THE EYE
ATLAS OF ANATOMICAL HISTORY

HÈCTOR BARAJAS M.

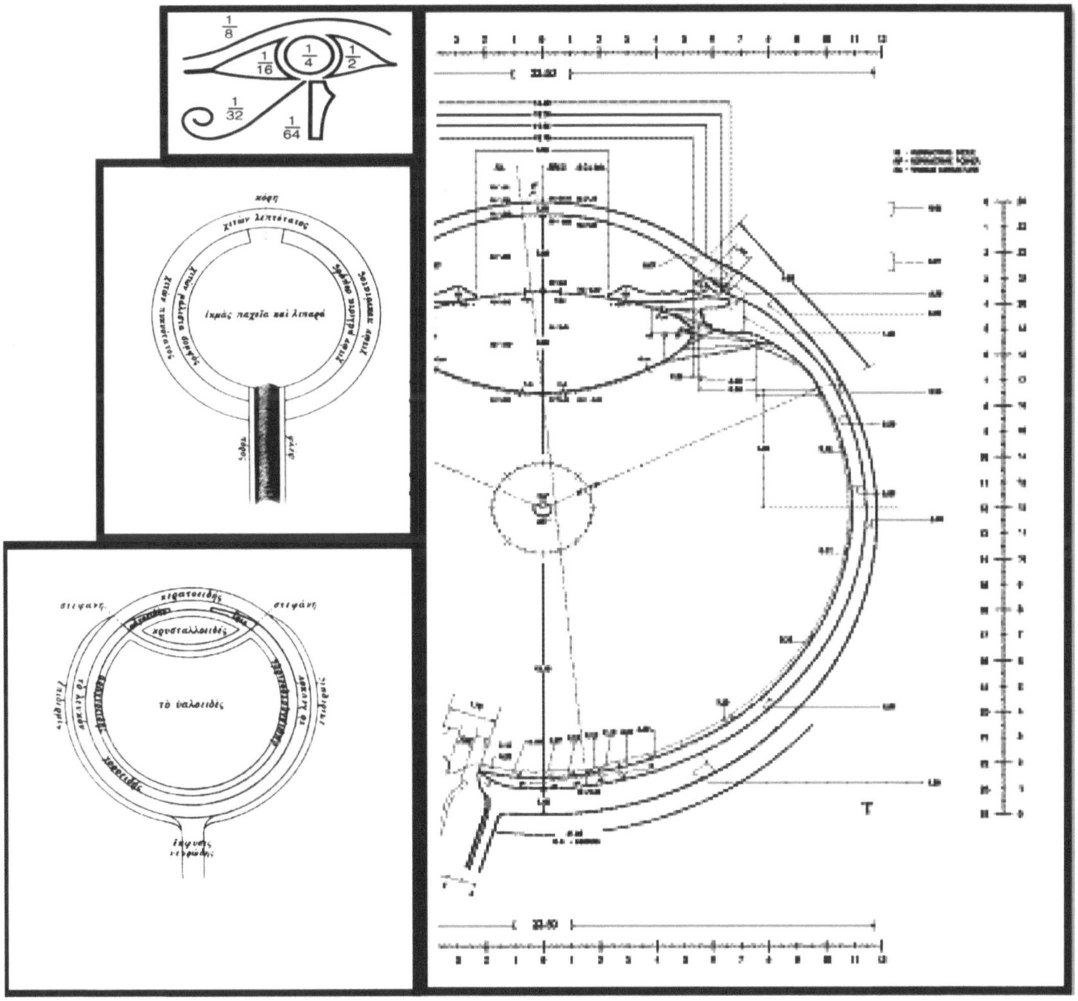

To order additional copies of this book, please contact:
Palibrio
1663 Liberty Drive
Suite 200
Bloomington, IN 47403
Toll Free from the U.S.A 877.407.5847
Toll Free from Mexico 01.800.288.2243
Toll Free from Spain 900.866.949
From other International locations +1.812.671.9757
Fax: 01.812.355.1576
orders@palibrio.com
419359

CONTENTS

THE EYE: ATLAS OF ANATOMICAL HISTORY

PURPOSE

INVESTIGATE THE EVOLUTION OF THE ANATOMICAL CHARACTERISTICS
OF THE EYE.

METHOD

BY MEANS OF THE ANALYSYS OF DISTINCT MEDICAL DOCUMENTS
THROUGH HISTORY, FROM THE EGYPTIANS, THE GREEKS, THE ROMANS,
THE ARABS, THE MIDDLE AGE, THE RENAISSANCE, UNTIL THE MODERNITY
AND CONTEMPORARIES.

RESULTS

THE ANATOMICAL CONCEPTS EVOLVED SINCE RUFO DE EFESO (98-117), A
MEDICAL GREEK THAT PERFORMED A PRECISE DESCRIPTION OF THE EYE
STRUCTURE, UNTIL SOEMMERRING (1775-1830) WHO DESCRIBED IN DETAIL
AN UP-TO-DATE ANATOMY OF THE EYE.

CONCLUSION

THE DESCRIPTION OF THE EYE ANATOMY HAS SUFFERED CONSTANT
AND REMARKABLE CHANGES, INFLUENCED BY THE METHODOLOGY AND
TECHNICAL ADVANCES APPLIED TO EYE RESEARCH ALONG THE HISTORY.

Domine, ut videam.
Lc 18:41

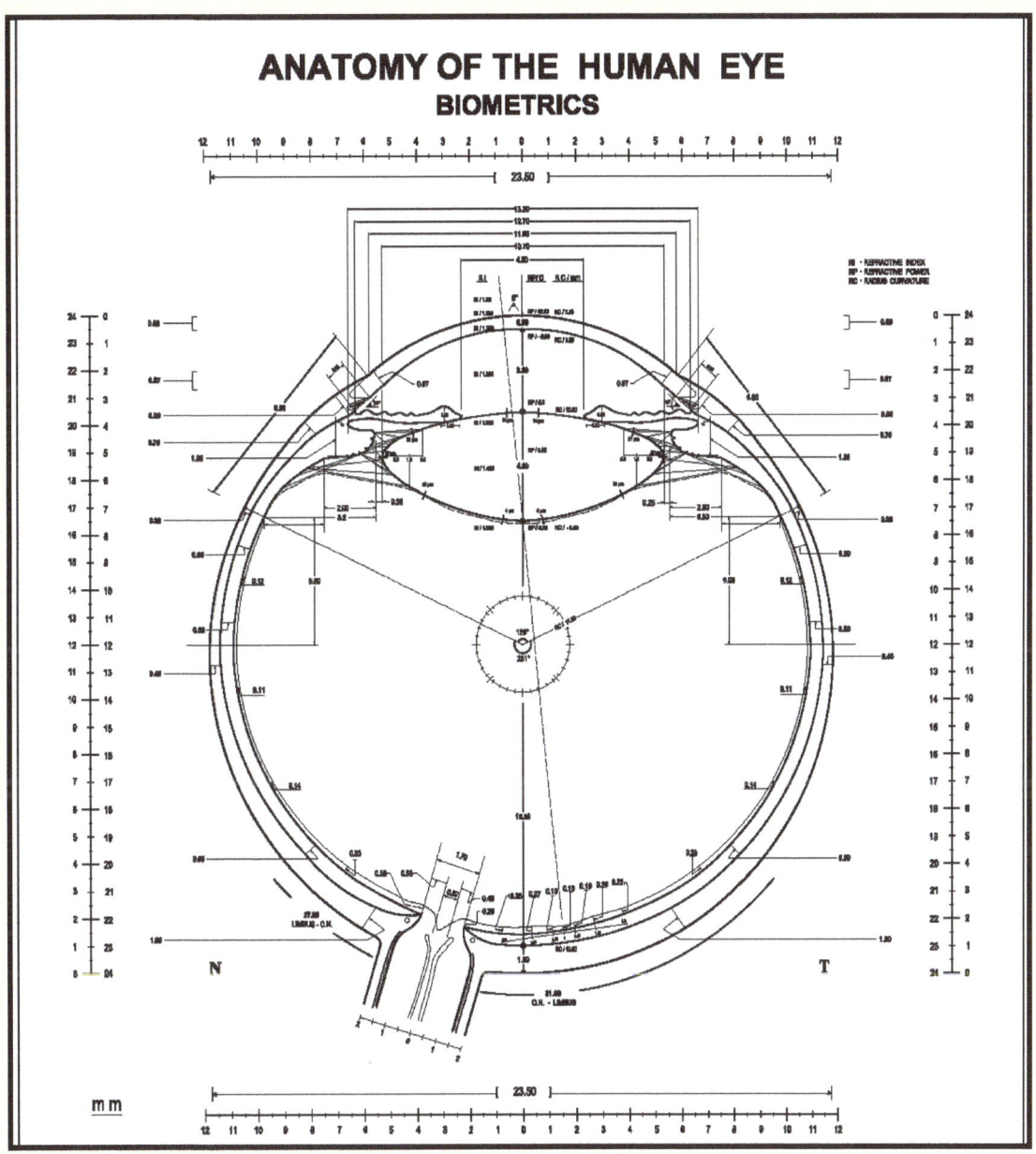

For an ophthalmologist, knowing the anatomic history of the eye is a passion, is searching in the depth of history the testimony of the most remote civilizations, of powerful and rich empires long gone by, to find the exquisite drawings that reveal to us the work of men of science that, overcoming their great limitations, delivered to us the description of human eye structure, as well as of the diseases that attacked it, including the medical and surgical treatments they used.

Some of this knowledge amazes us because it is still valid. The time devoted to this work has allowed me to enjoy yet another aspect of ophthalmology, when I contemplate the marvelous product of men of science, that in a common interest, carried out research, joined efforts and described to us the anatomy of the vision organ through history.

The collection is incomplete: there are new archaeological and bibliographical discoveries every single day, and I will continue to look for them. This is just the beginning and a modest recognition of the persons who have contributed to describing the eye.

I invite you to start a journey through the history of science and become acquainted with the graphic evolution of the anatomic and physiological concept of the eye globe by regions and ages of humankind.

The interest in knowing the secrets of human body, particularly the eye, is evident since the time of the Egyptian pharaohs (2400 B.C.) with the first ophthalmologist known in medical history: Pepi Ankh Or Iri.

In the amazing Babylon where King Hammurabi established professional practice standards in 1800 B.C. In the India of Susruta, in the Greece of Democritus, Hippocrates and Aristotle.

In Alexandria, we find the anatomists Herophilus of Chalcedon and Erasistratus of Chios.

In the Imperial Rome, we have Claudius Galenus of Pergamum and Pedanius Dioscorides.

In the Arabian medicine, we have Avicenna, of Hunayn ibn Ishaq, Averroes, and Alhazen.

The same interest continued during the Middle Age, when science became secret, enriched itself and was divulged only in monasteries.

During this time, the great contributions were made by the Benedictine monk Constantinus Africanus in Salerno; Gerardo de Cremona in Toledo; the Portuguese Petrus Hispanicus, a traveling doctor who later became Pope John XXI; and the Franciscan monk Roger Bacon in England.

During the splendor of the Renaissance, Leonardo da Vinci, George Bartich, Chistophorus Scheiner, Hieronymus Fabricius Acuapendente, and Andreas Vesalius stand out for their anatomic and physiological knowledge.

Centuries later, this work was continued by Renatus Descartus, Isaac Newton, Claude Nicolás le Cat, Johann Gott Fried Zinn, Samuel T. Von Soemmerring, Joan Esperson Weddel, illustrator of the work by Jorge A. Alvarado and Michael J. Hogan.

The anatomic history of the eye was found and rescued following the line of time. Sculptures, papyrus, codices, manuscripts, incunabula, unique editions were reviewed to prepare this work.
I thank my professors, my friends and the staff of the libraries and museums that allowed me to search through their archives.

H.B.

Para el mêdico oftalmòlogo. Conocer la historia anatómica del ojo, es una pasión, es buscar entre las profundidades de la historia , los testimonios de las civilizaciones màs remotas , de poderosos y ricos imperios ya desaparecidos, encontrando los dibujos exquisitos que nos revelan el trabajo de los hombres de ciencia que, en medio de grandes limitaciones se imponen y nos entregan la descripción de la estructura del ojo humano así como las enfermedades que le afligen, los tratamientos médicos y quirúrgicos de cada época. Algunos de estos conocimientos nos asombran por su vigencia.

El tiempo dedicado a esta obra me ha permitido disfrutar un aspecto más de la oftalmología, al contemplar el producto maravilloso del trabajo de los hombres de ciencia, que en un interés común, realizan sus investigaciones, suman esfuerzos y nos describen la anatomia del organo de la visiòn a travès de la historia

La colección es incompleta: cada día existen nuevos descubrimientos arqueologicos y bibliográficos, seguiremos buscando. Esto solo es el inicio y un modesto reconocimiento a las personas que han contribuido a describir el órgano de la visión.

Iniciemos un viaje en la historia de la ciencia y conoceremos, por regiones y etapas de la humanidad, la evolución grafica del concepto anatómico y fisiológico del globo ocular.

El interés por conocer los secretos del cuerpo humano, en particular del ojo, se muestra desde la epoca de los faraones de de Egipto -2 400 A.C.- con el primer oftalmólogo conocido en la historia medica.

-Pepi Ankh Or Iri-

En la deslumbrante Babilonia donde el rey Hammurabi, establece las normas de la práctica profesional, 1 800 A.C.

En la India de Susruta, en la Grecia de Democritus, de Hipócrates, de Aristoteles.

En Alejandría, los anatomistas Herophilus de Chalcedonia y Erasistratus de Chíos.

En la Roma imperial de Claudius Galenus de Pergamo, de Dioscórides de Pedaníus.

En la medicina arabe de Avicena, de Hunain ibn Ishak, de Averroes, de Alhazen.

El mismo interês continua durante la edad media, cuando la ciencia se guarda, se enriquece y se difunde en los monasterios.

Durante esta época las grandes aportaciones las realizan, el monje benedictino Constantinus Africanus, en Salerno. Gerardo de Cremona en Toledo. El lucitano Petrus Hispanicus médico itinerante conocido como S.S. Juan XXI. El monje franciscano Roger Bacon en Inglaterra. En el esplendor del renacimiento destacan por sus conocimientos anatómicos y fisiológicos Leonardo da Vinci, George Bartich, Chistophorus Scheiner, Hieronymus Fabricius Acuapendente, Andreas Vesalius. Siglos después continuaran esta obra Renatus Descartus, Isaac Newton, Claude Nicolâs le Cat, Johann Gott Fried Zinn, Samuel T. Von Soemmerring y Joan Esperson Weddel, illustrador de la obra de Jorge A. Alvarado y Michael J.Hogan

La historia anatómica del ojo fue encontrada y rescatada siguiendo la lînea del tiempo. Se revisaron esculturas, papiros, códices, manuscritos, libros incunables, ediciones ùnicas.
Mi agradecimiento a mis maestros, a mis amigos así como al personal de las bibliotecas y de los museos que me permitieron buscar en sus archivos .

H.B

Egypt
2600 BC

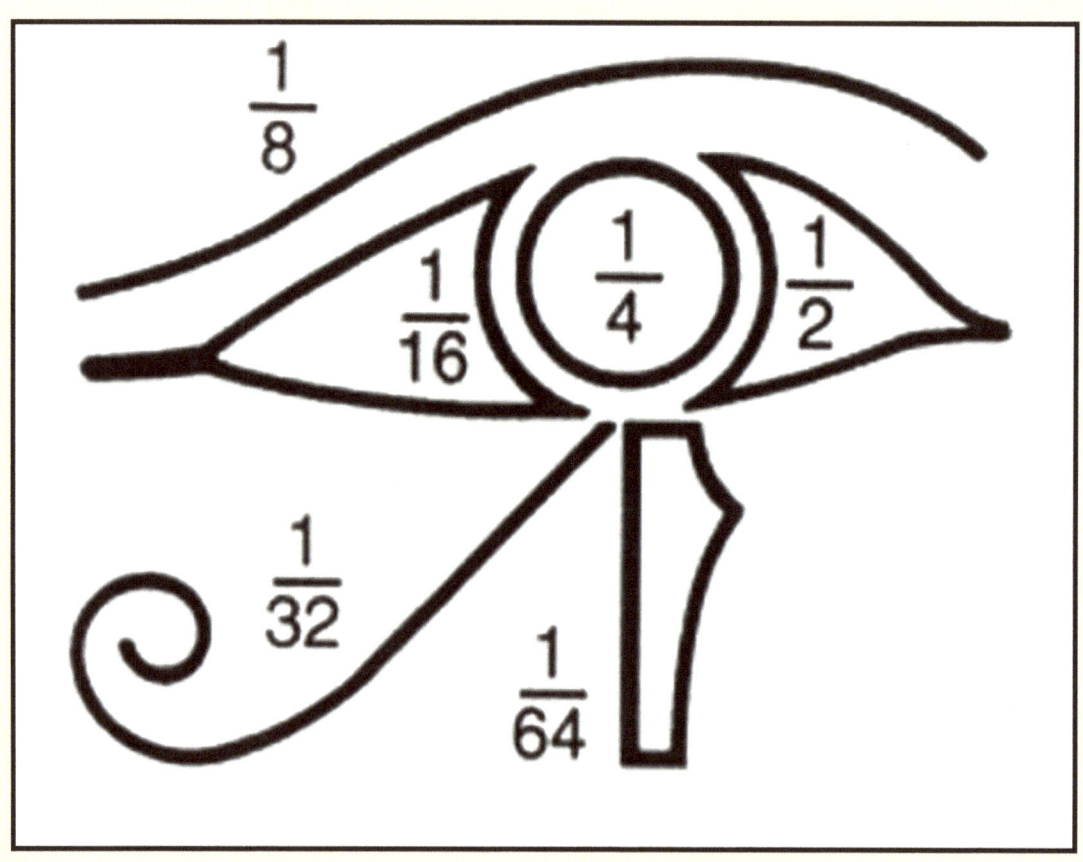

Greece

Democritus of Abdera

-

Hippocrates of Cos

-

Aristotle of Stegira

-

Herophilos of Chalcedon

-

Erasistratus of Cos

Greece

Democritus of Abdera
470 – 380.

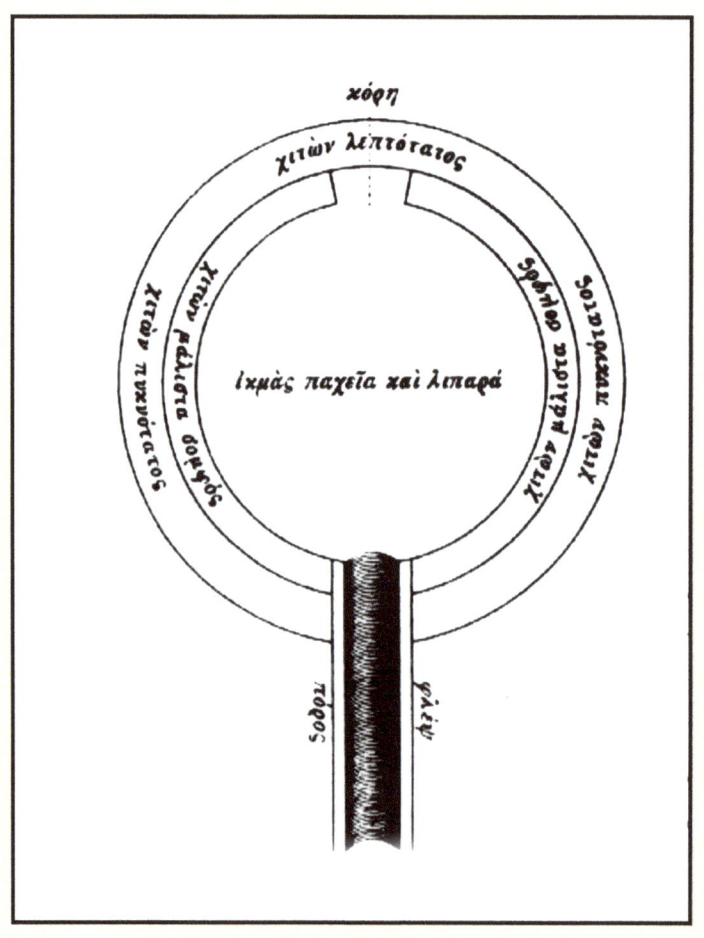

Greece

Hippocrates of Cos
460 – 370
Opus:
Medicorum Omnium Princips

* * *

Aristotle of Stagira
384 – 322
Opus:
De Physicae Auscultationis

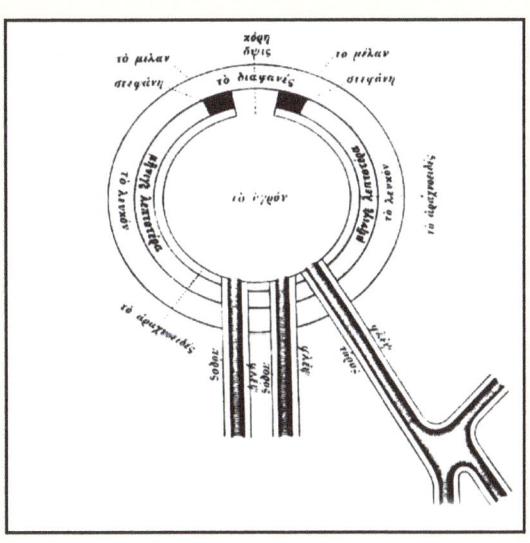

Alexandria

Herophilos of Chalcedon
300 – 250
Erasistratus of Cos
304 – 250

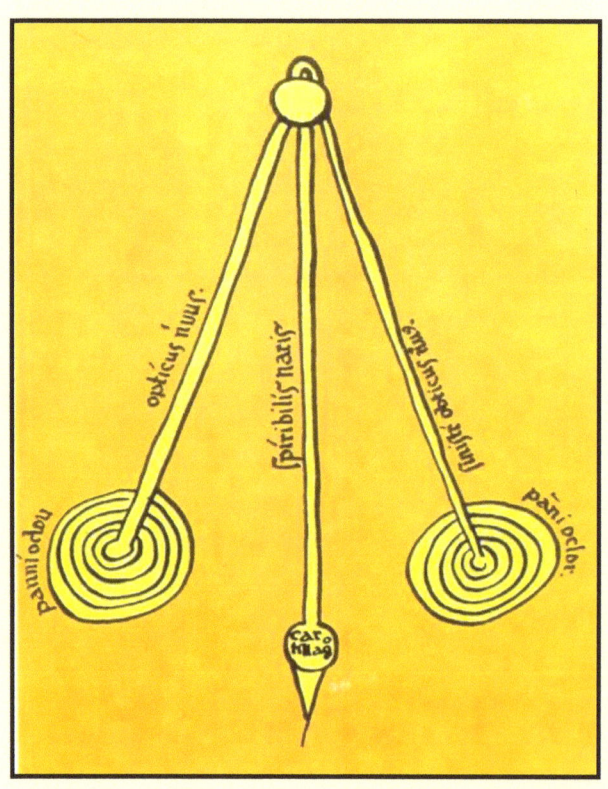

Rome

Aulus Cornelius Celsus

\-

Rufus of Ephesus

\-

Claudius Galenus of Pergamon

Rome

Aulus Cornelius Celsus
25 – 50
Opus:
In hoc volumine haec continentur
De Medicina Libri Octo

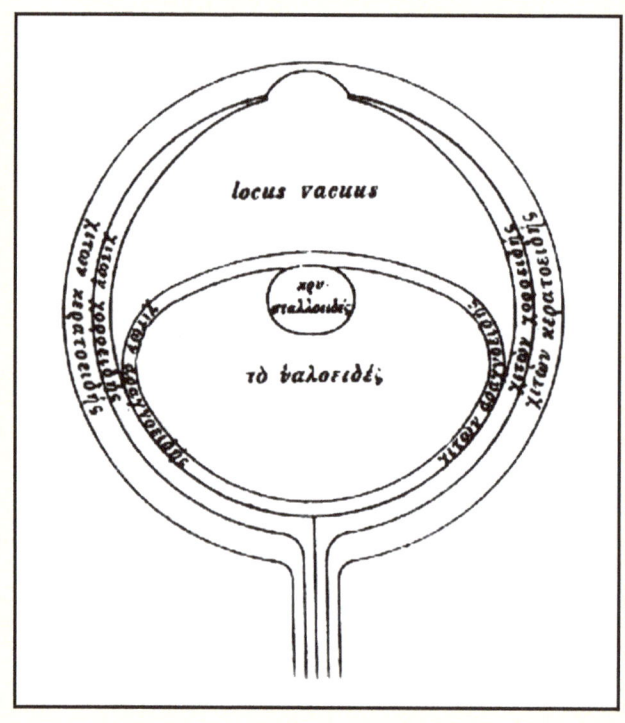

Rome

Rufus of Ephesus
98 – 117
Opus:
Anatomia Oculus
de vesicae renumque morbis
de purgantibus medicamentis
de partibus corporis humani.
cornea, conjuntiva, lens cristalinus,
corpus vitrens, quiasun opticus.

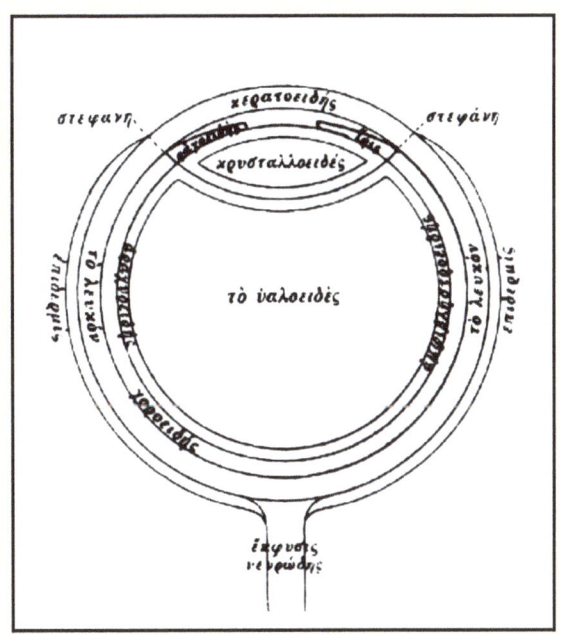

Rome

Claudius Galenus of Pergamum
130 – 200
Opus:
Ars Medicinalis
De ratione curandi ad
Glauconem
Terapeutica
Definitiones rarum medicarum

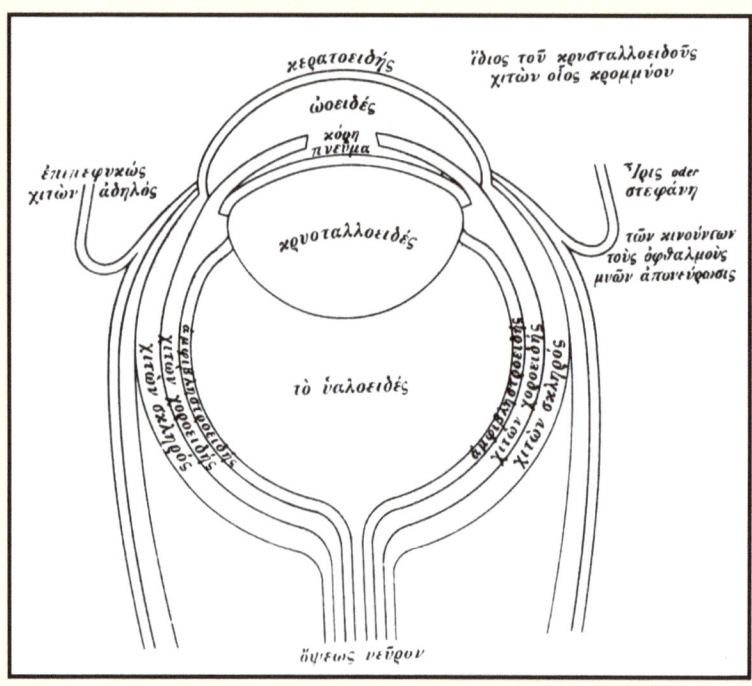

Arabs

Hunain ibu Ishar

-

Alhazen Ibn al-Haitham

-

Abu'Ali Ibn Sina Alhusayn
Ibn ABD allah
Avicena

-

Alcoati of Toledo

-

Haile Halif Ben Ali

-

Tanquih al Manazir

-

Abu' l Hassan Al Farsi

Arabs

Hunain ibn Ishar
809–873
Opus:
Book of the Ten Treatises on the Eye

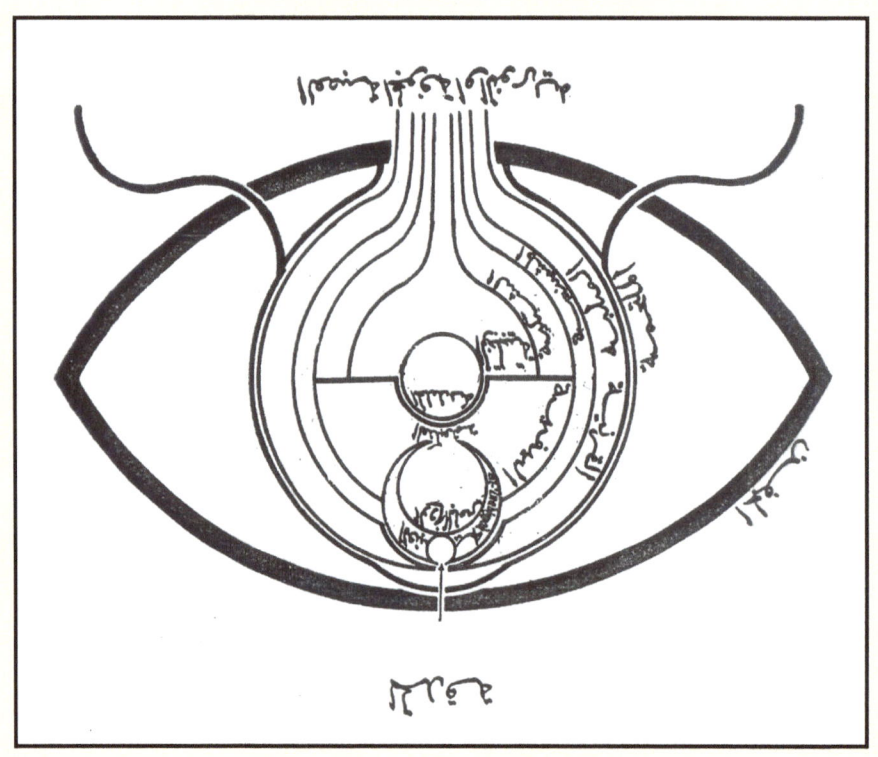

Arabs

Alhazen   Ibn al Haitam
965 – 1039
Opus:
Peri   Optices
Opticae   Thesaurus

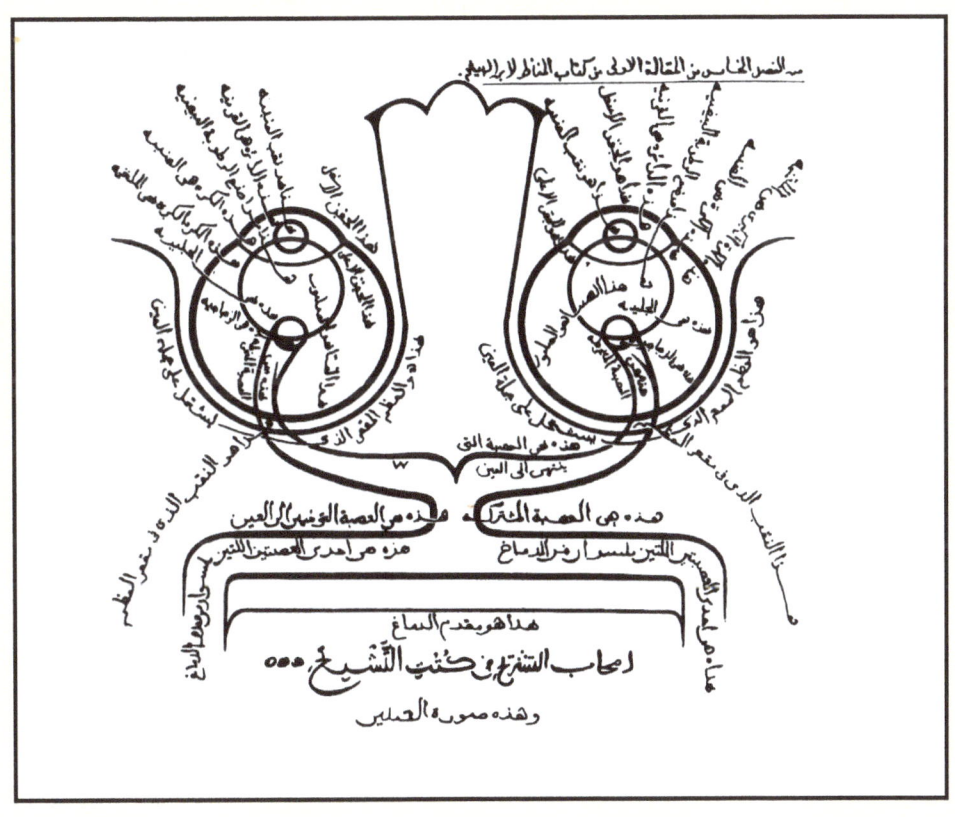

Arabs

Alhazen   Ibn al Haitam
965 – 1039
Opus:
Peri   Optices
Opticae   Thesaurus

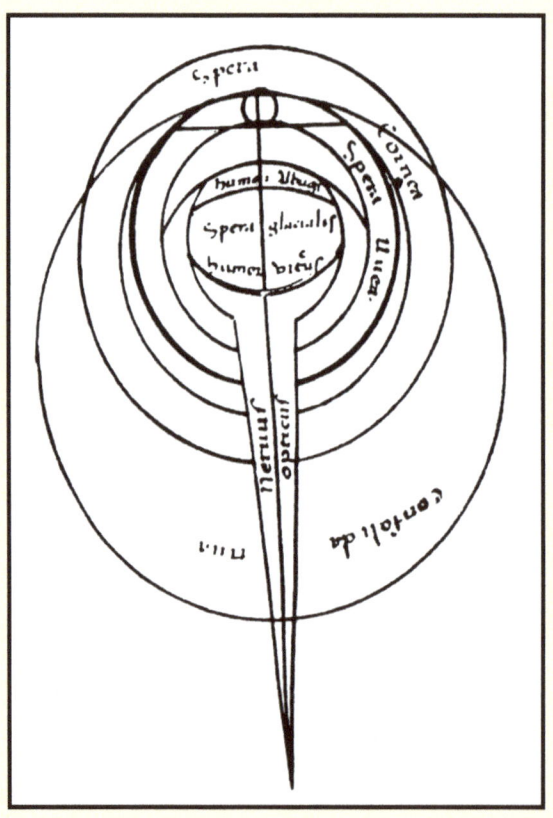

Arabs

Alhazen   Ibn al Haitam
965 – 1039
Opticae Thesaurus

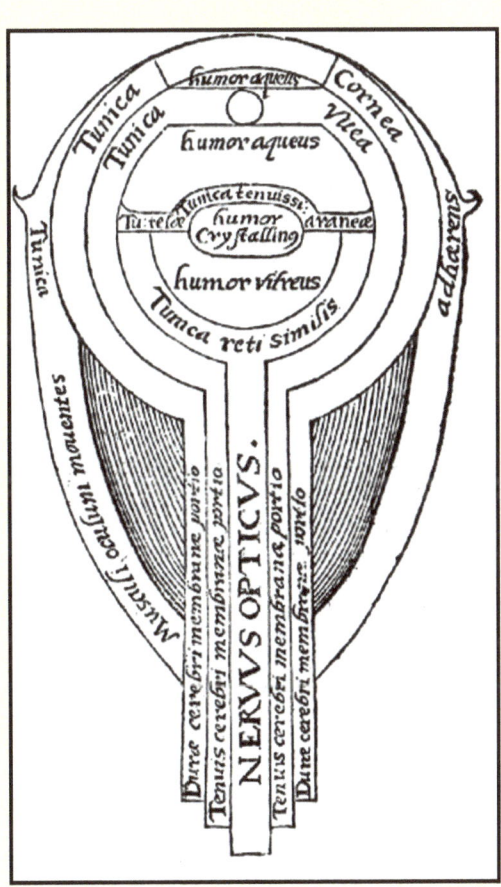

Arabs

Abu´ Ali ibn Sina Alhusayn ibnABDAllah
-Avicena-
980 – 1037
Opus:
Cannon Medicinae

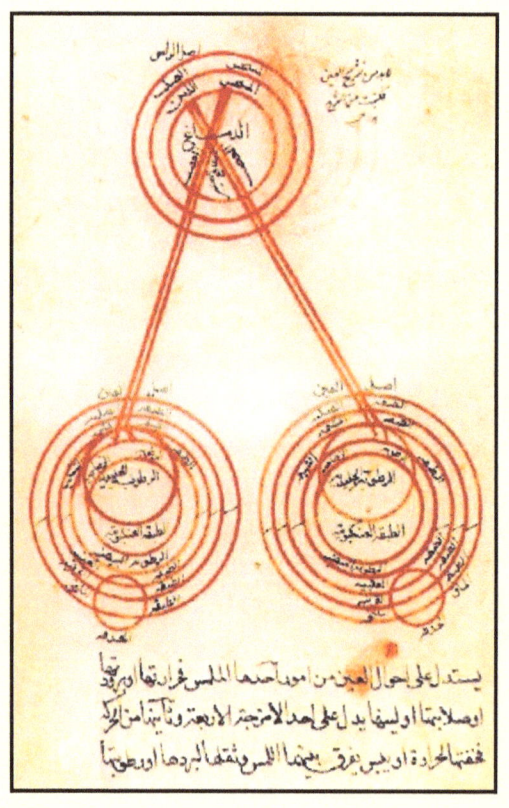

Arabs

Alcoati of Toledo
1160
Opus:
Liber de Oculis

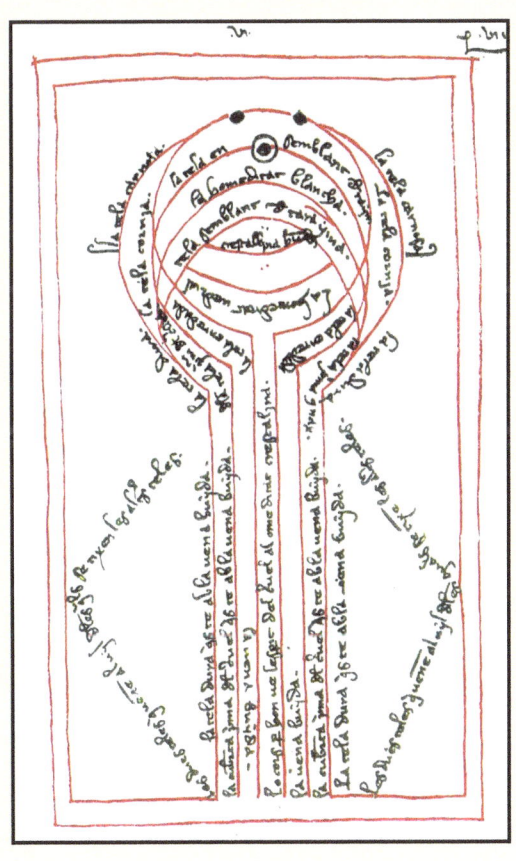

Arabs

Haile Halif Ben Ali
1266

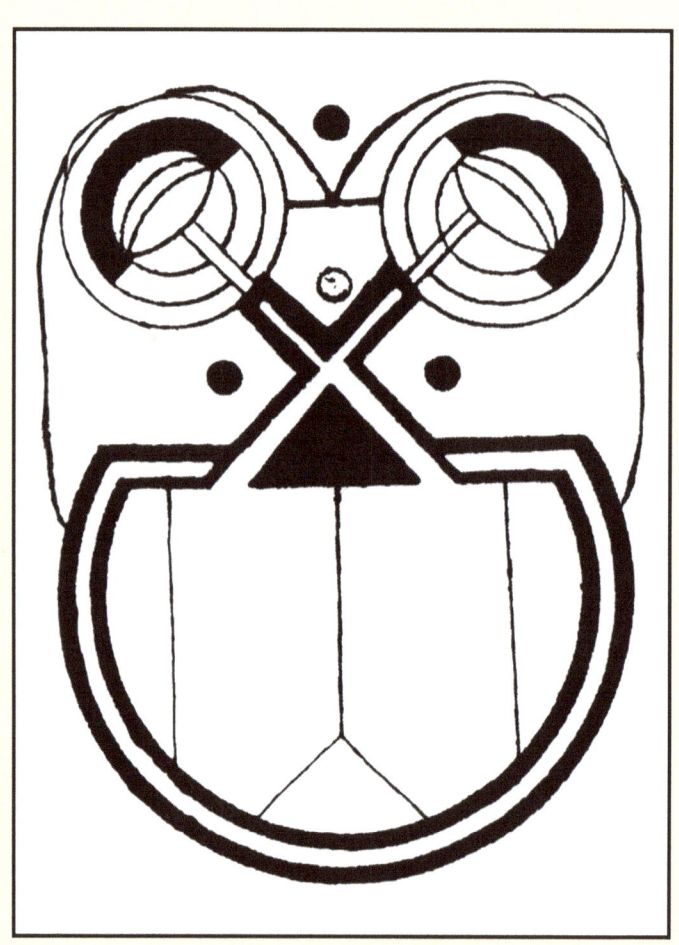

Arabs

Tanquih al Manazir
1316

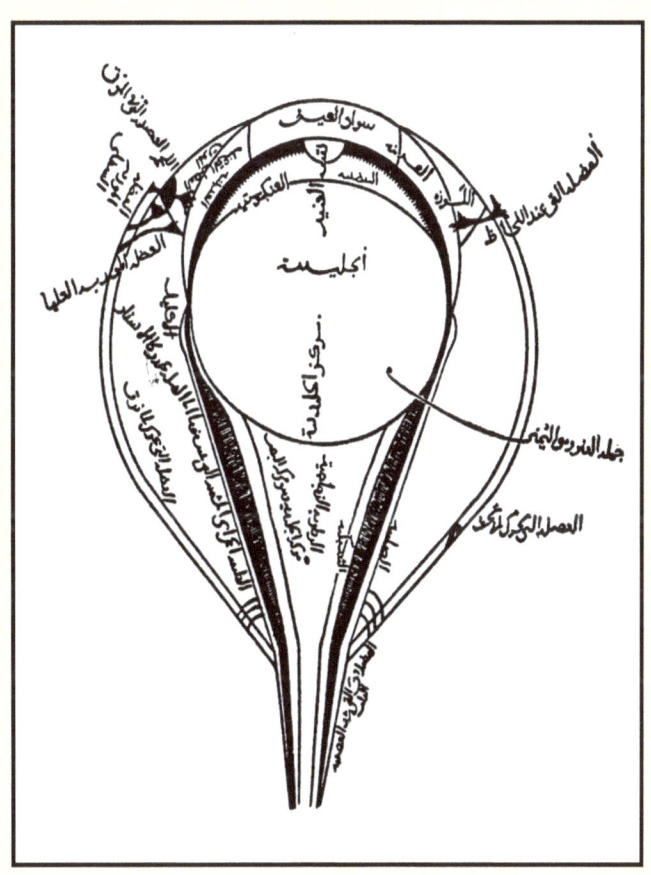

Arabs

Abu 'l Hassan Al Farsi
1443

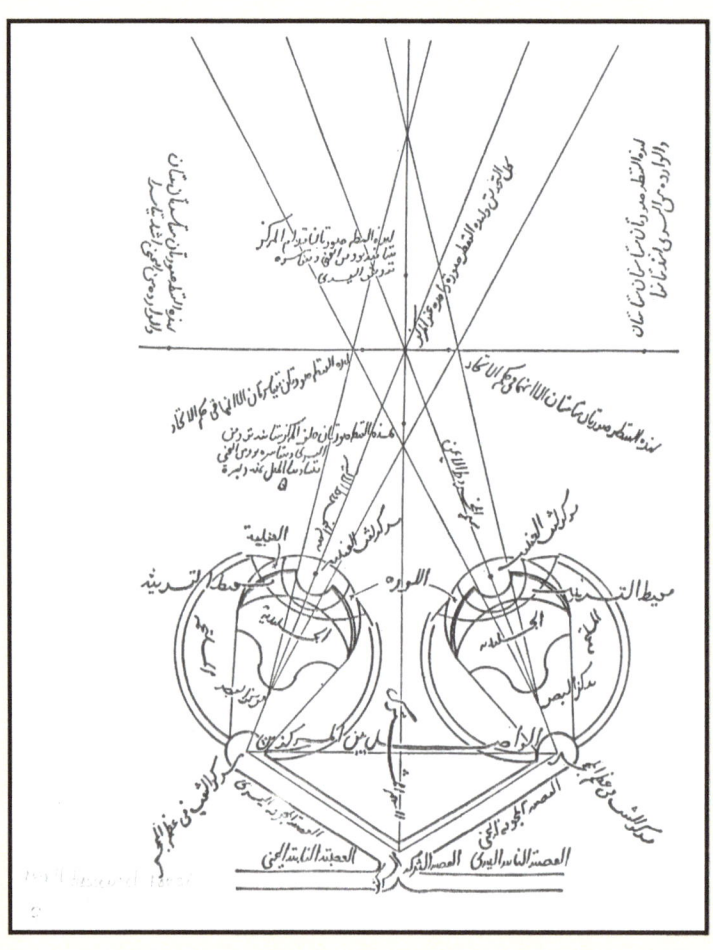

Middle Age

John Peckham - Roger Bacon - Witelio

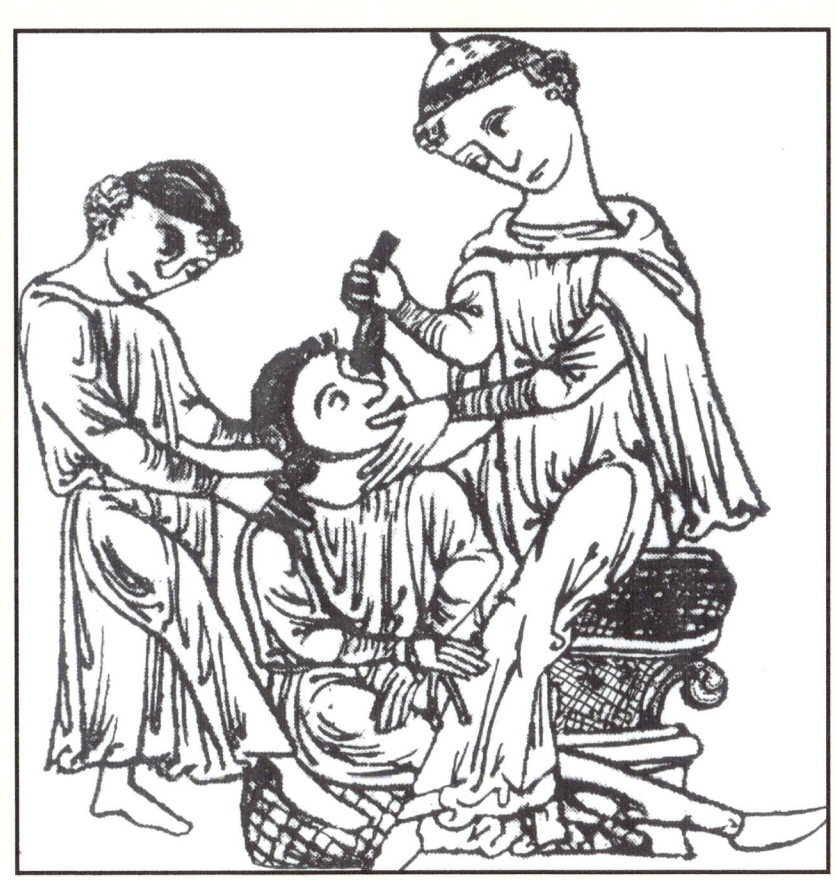

Middle Age

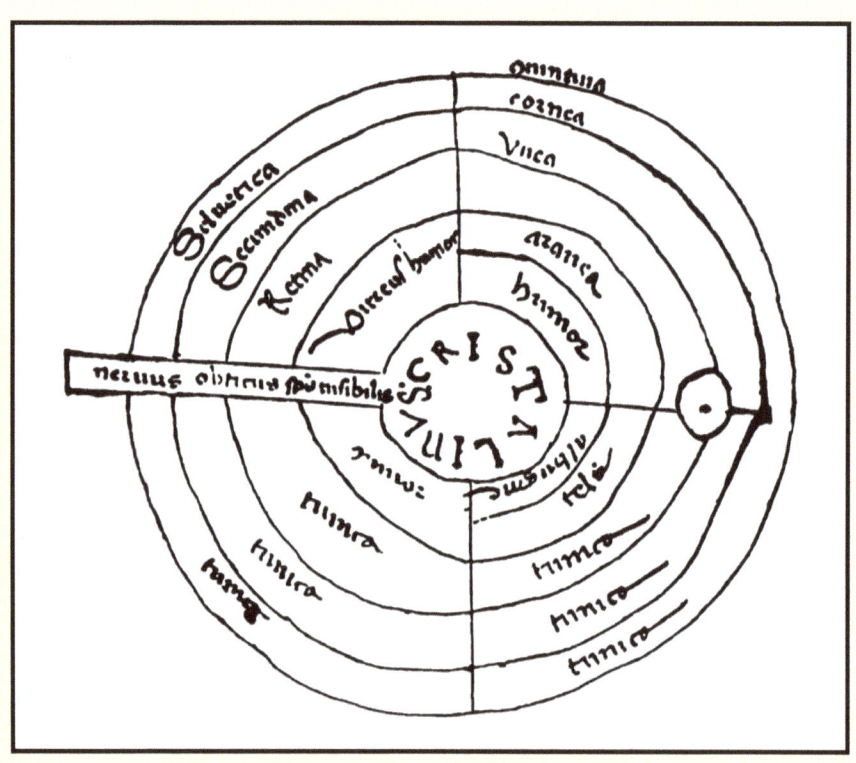

Middle Age

John Peckham
1230 – 1292
Opus:
Perspectiva communis
Onmibus philosophiae
Studiosis necessaria

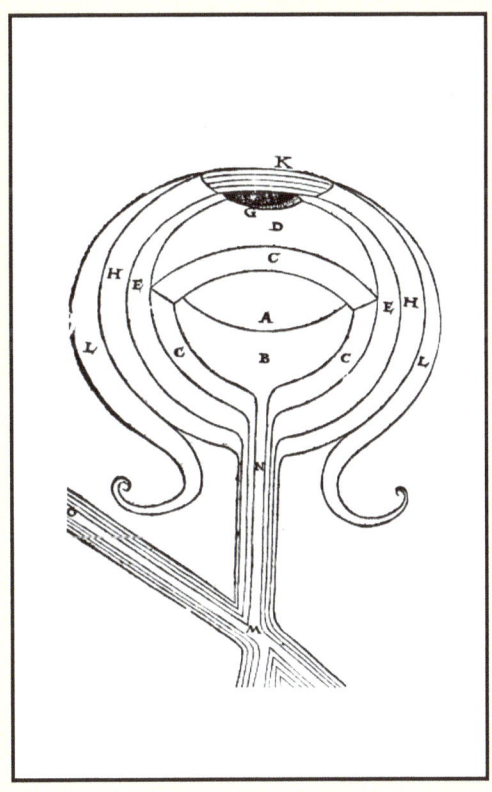

Middle Age

Roger Bacon
1214 – 1294
Opus:
Opus Maius

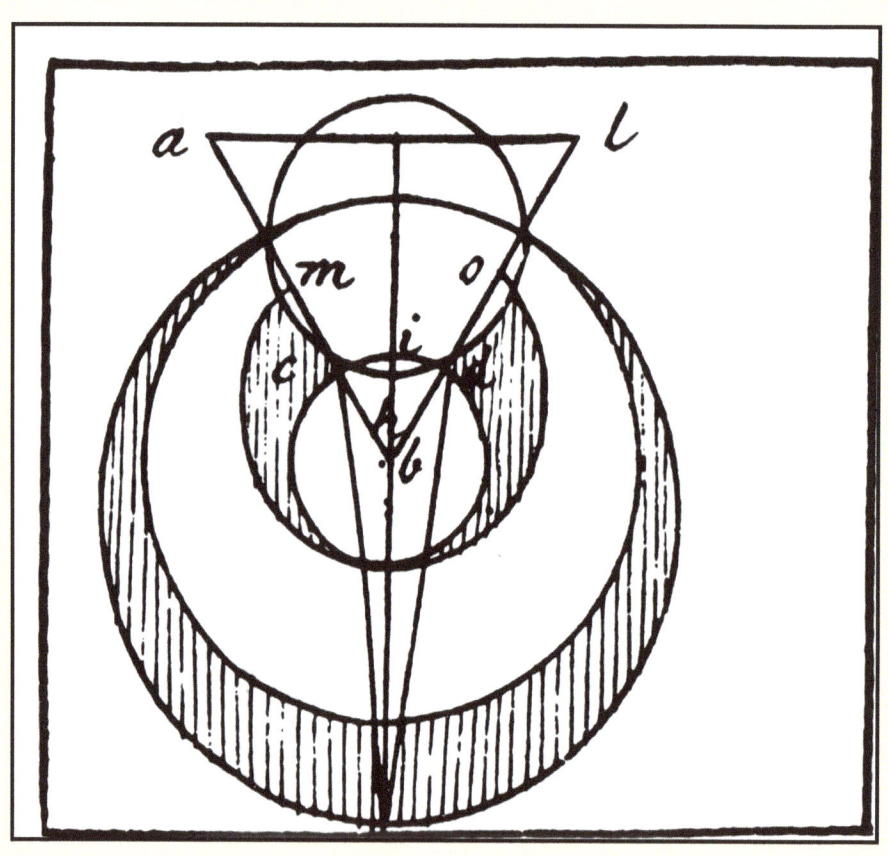

Middle Age

Witelio
1230 – 1275
Opus:
Peri Optikes

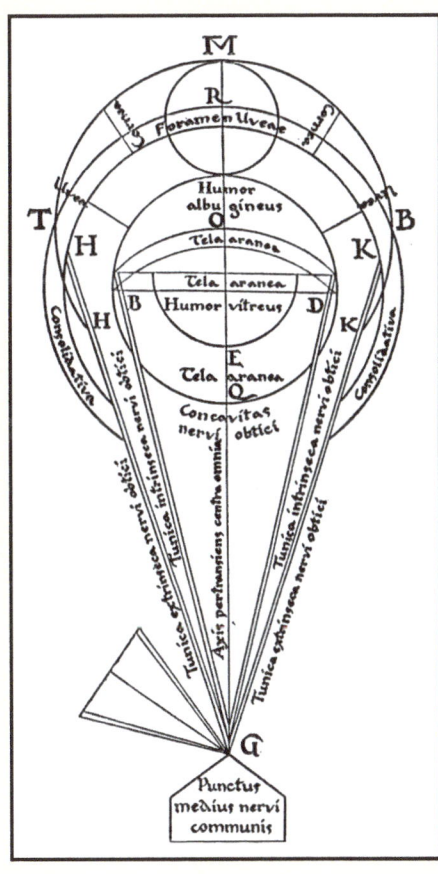

Renaissance

Leonardo da Vinci

-

Francesco Maurolico

-

Leonheart Fuchs

-

Georg Bartich

-

Hieronimus Fabricius A.B. Aquapendente

-

Andreas Vesalius

-

Cornelius Gemma

Renaissance

Leonardo da Vinci
1452 - 1519

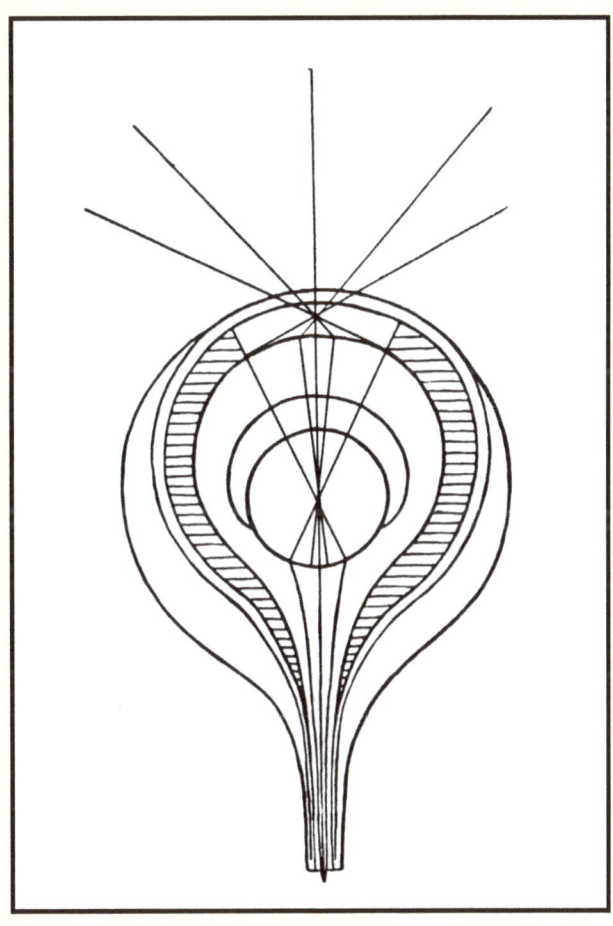

Renaissance

Francesco Maurolico
1494-1575
Opus :
Phostisimi de lumine et ubra

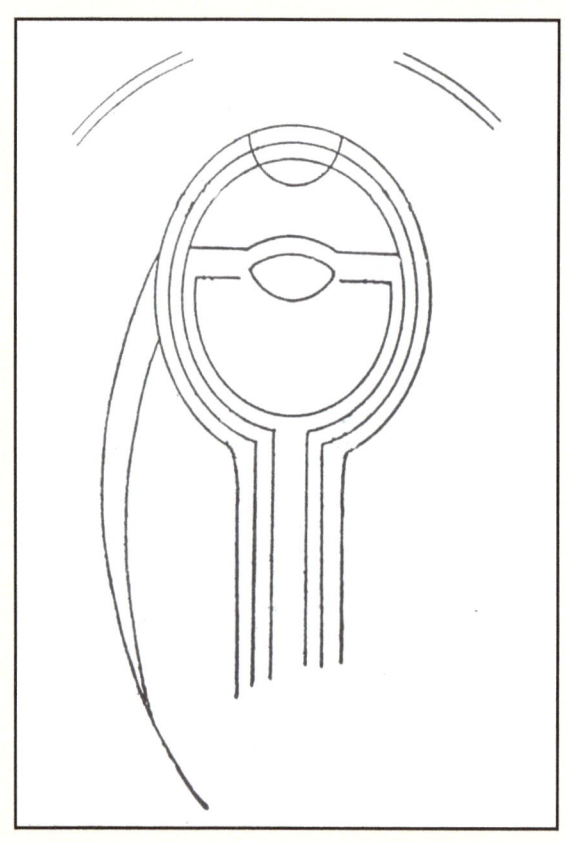

Renaissance

Leonheart Fuchs
1501 – 1566
Opus:
Tabula oculorum morbos comprehendens
De curandi Ratione
Alle Kraunckheyt der Augen

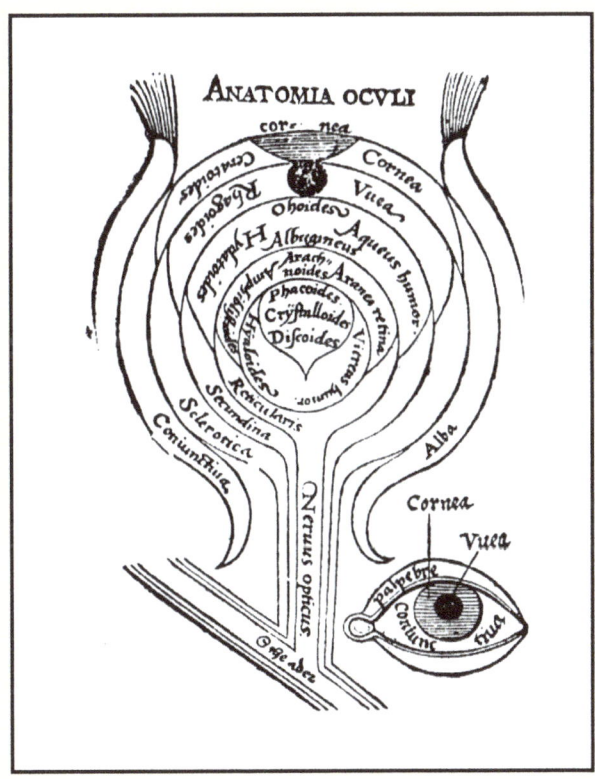

Renaissance

Georg Bartich
1535 – 1606
Opus:
Ophthalmoduleia Das ist augendienst

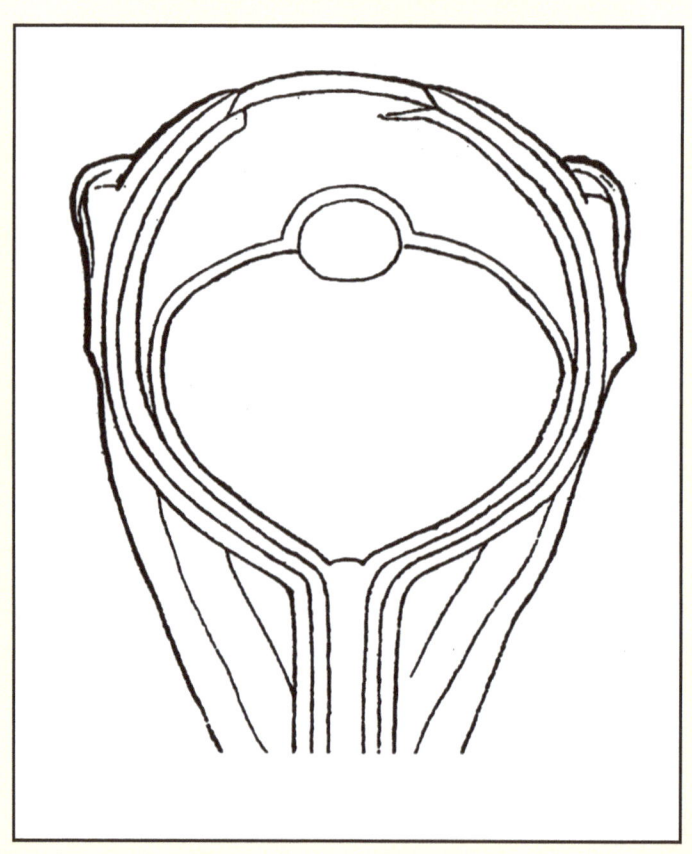

Renaissance

Hieronymus Fabricius A.B. Aquapendente
1537 – 1619
Opus:
De visione, voce, auditu
tractatus anatomicus triplex, quorum
primns de oculo
Oeures Chirurgicales

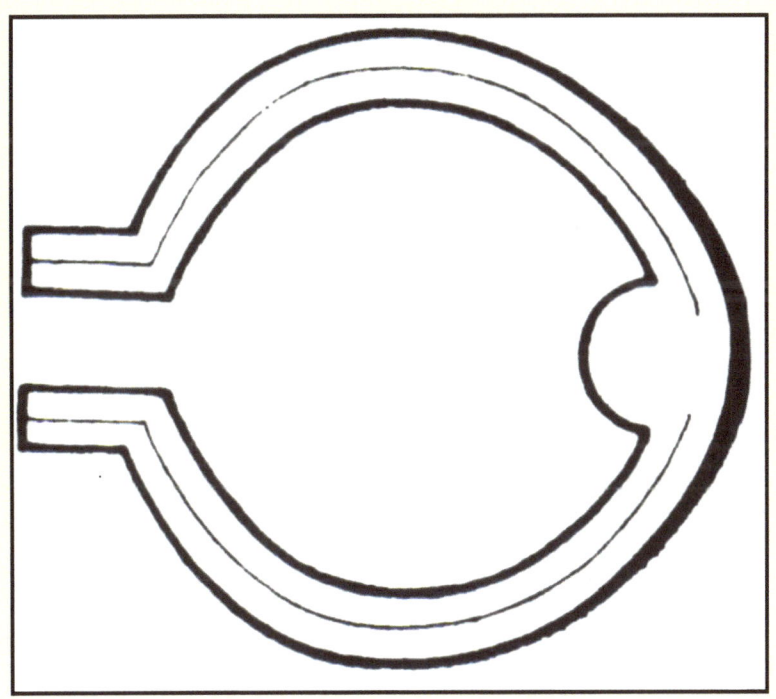

Renaissance

Andreas Vesalius
1514 – 1564
Opus:
De Humani Corporis Fábrica

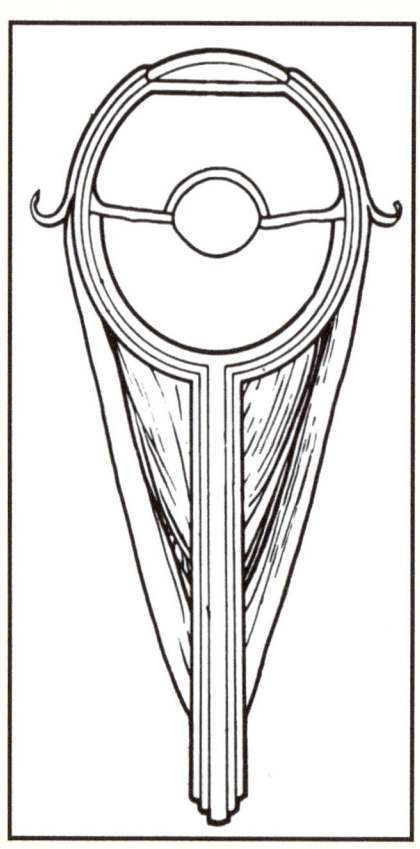

Renaissance

Cornelius Gemma
1535 – 1579
De arte cyclognomica

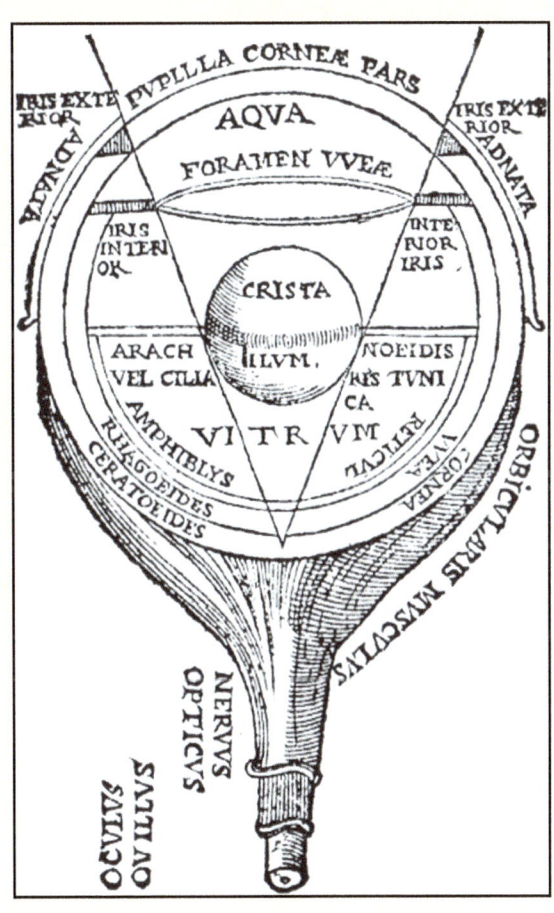

Christophorus Scheiner
1575 – 1650
Opus:
Oculus hoc est: fundamentum Opticum
In quo ex accurata oculi

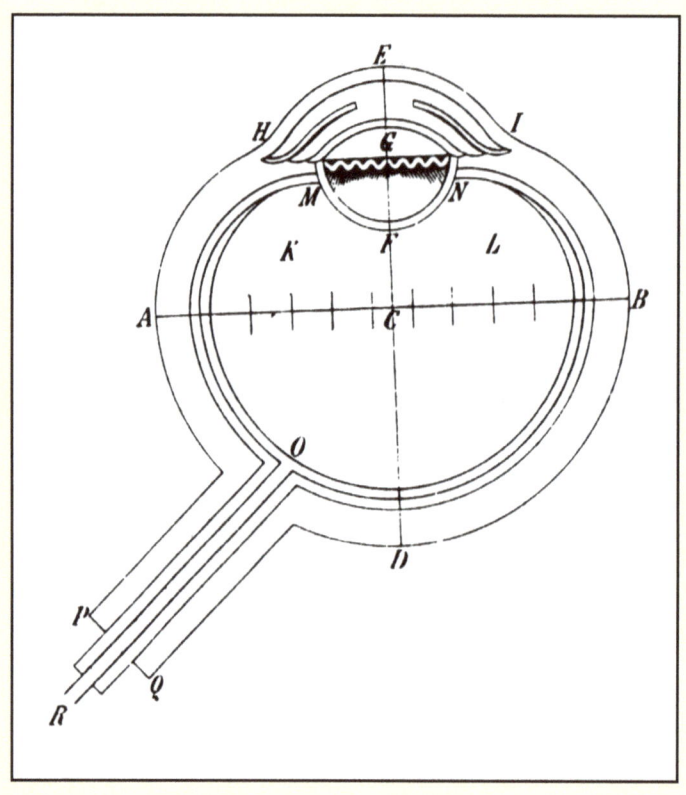

S.XVI-XVII

Renatus Descartus
1596 – 1650
Opus:
Dioptrice
l´Homme
Principia Philosophiae

S.XVII-XVIII

William Briggs
1642 – 1704
Opus:
Ophthalmo – graphia
sive oculi ejusque partium
descriptio anatomica

S.XVII-XVIII

Isaac Newton
1642 – 1727
Opus:
Principia   Mathematica

S.XVIII

Claude Nicolas le Cat
1700 – 1768
Opus:
Traite des Sens
A Physiacal essay on the senses

S.XVIII

John Taylor
1703 – 1772
Opus:
An account of the mechanism

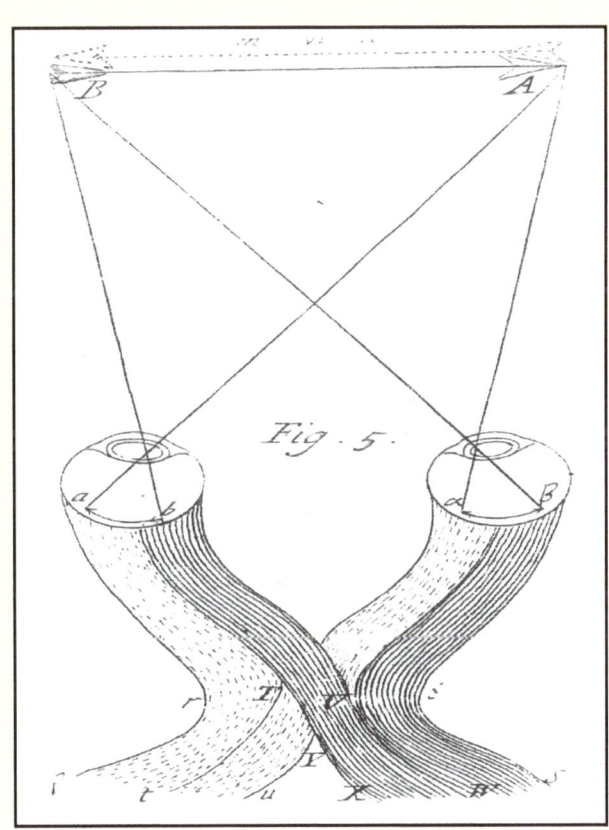

S.XVIII

Johann Gott Fried Zinn
1727 – 1759
Opus:
Descriptio Anatomica Oculi
Humani Iconibus Ilustrata

S. XVIII-XIX

Samuel T. Von Soemmerring
1755 – 1830
Opus:
Icones Oculi Humani

S. XX

Michael J. Hogan
Jorge A. Alvarado
Joan Esperson Weddell

Opus:
Histology of the human eye

W.B. Saunders company 1971

Greece

Democritus of Abdera 470 – 380.

Hippocrates of Cos 460 – 370

**

Aristotle of Stagira 384 – 322

Herophilos of Chalcedon 300 – 250

Erasistratus of Cos 304 – 250

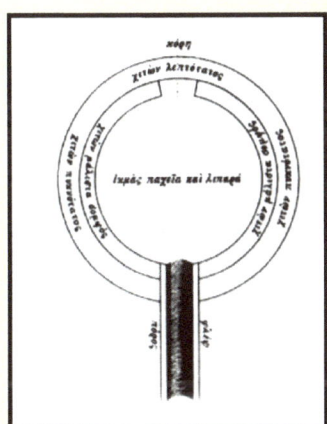

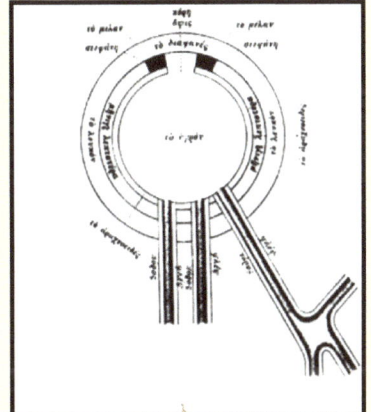

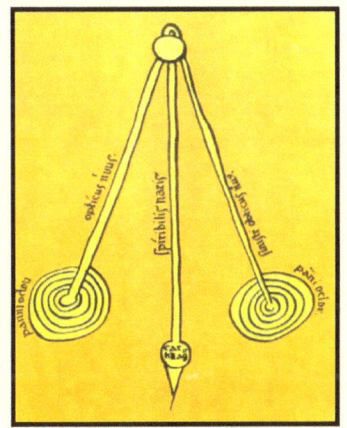

Rome

Aulus Cornelius Celsus 25 – 50

Rufus of Ephesus 98 – 117

Galenus of Pergamum 130 – 200

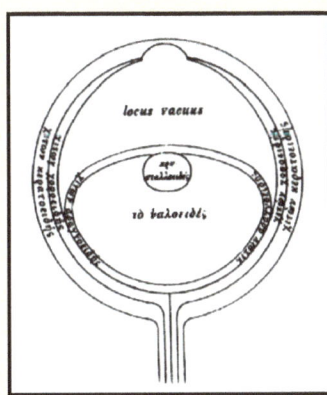

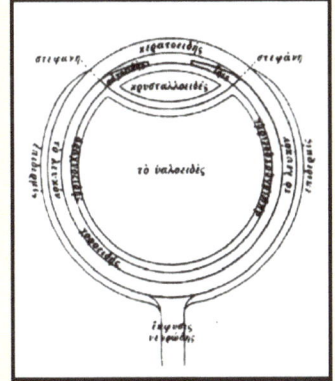

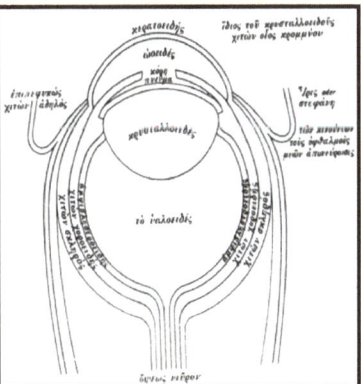

Arabs

Abu´ Ali ibn Sina -Avicena-
980 – 1037

Alcoati of Toledo
1160

Hunain ibu Ishar
809–873

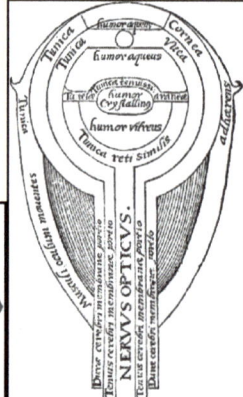

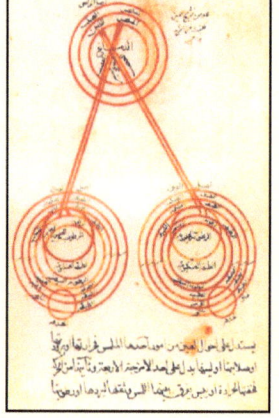

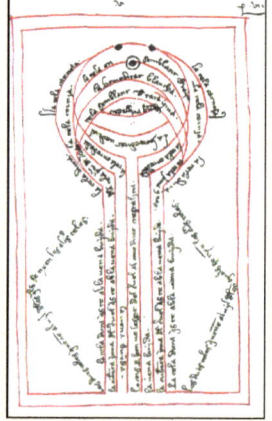

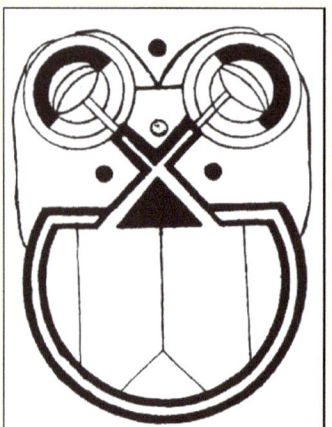

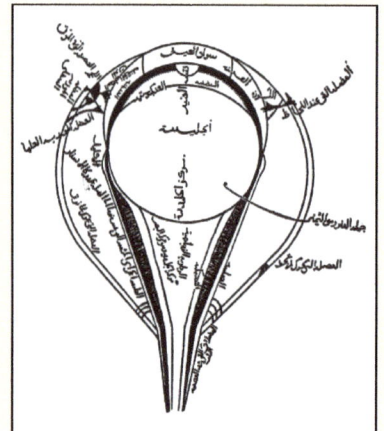

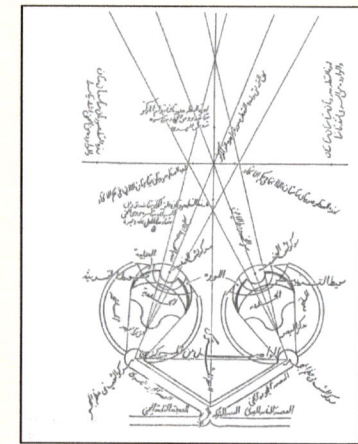

Tanquih al Manazir
Abul Hasan
1316

Tanquih al Manazir
Abul Hasan
1316

Abu´l Hassan Al Farsi
1443

Middle Age

Codex Trivultianus

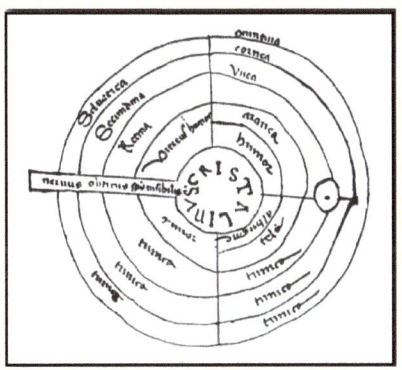

John Peckham
1230 – 1292

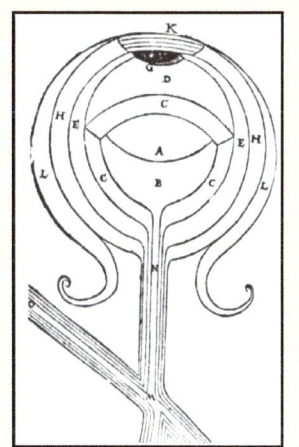

Witelio
1230 – 1275

Roger Bacon
1214 – 1294

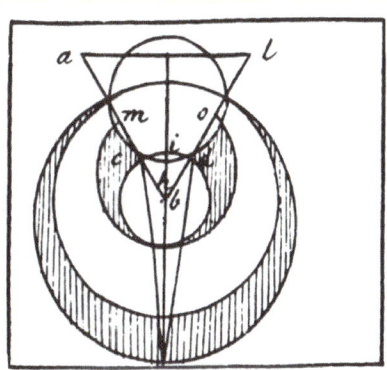

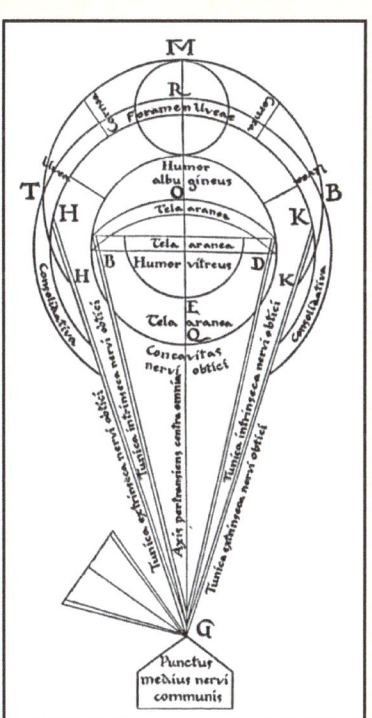

Renaissance

**Hieronymus Fabricius A.B. Aquapendente
1537 – 1619**

**Leonardo da Vinci
1452 - 1519**

**Leonheart Fuchs
1501 – 1566**

**Andreas Vesalius
1514 – 1564**

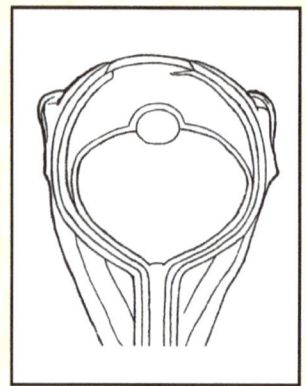

**Georg Bartich
1535 – 1606**

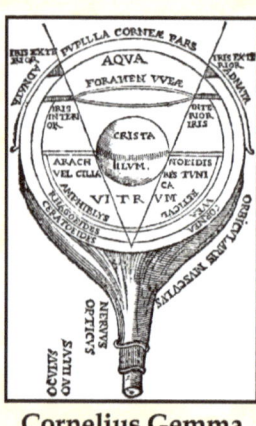

**Cornelius Gemma
1535 – 1579**

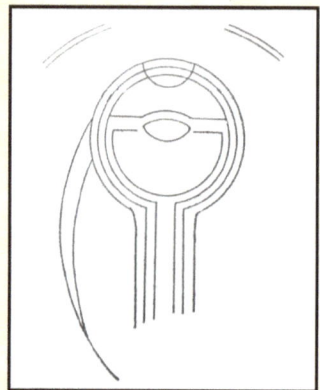

**Francesco Maurolico
1494-1575**

Christophorus Scheiner
1575 – 1650

Renatus Descartus
1596 – 1650

William Briggs
1642 – 1704

Isaac Newton
1642 – 1727

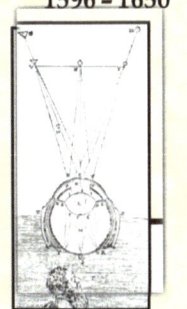

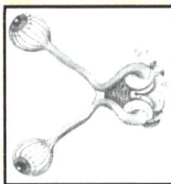

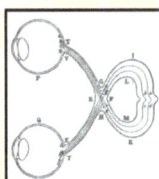

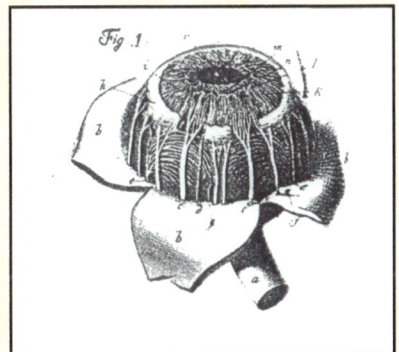

Johann Gott Fried Zinn
1727 – 1759

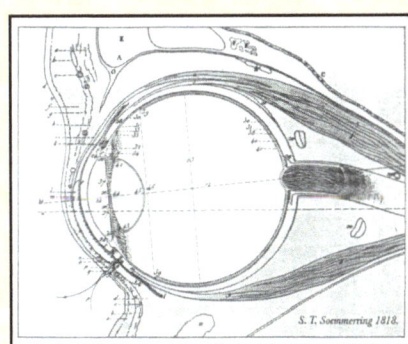

Samuel T. Von Soemmerring
1755 – 1830

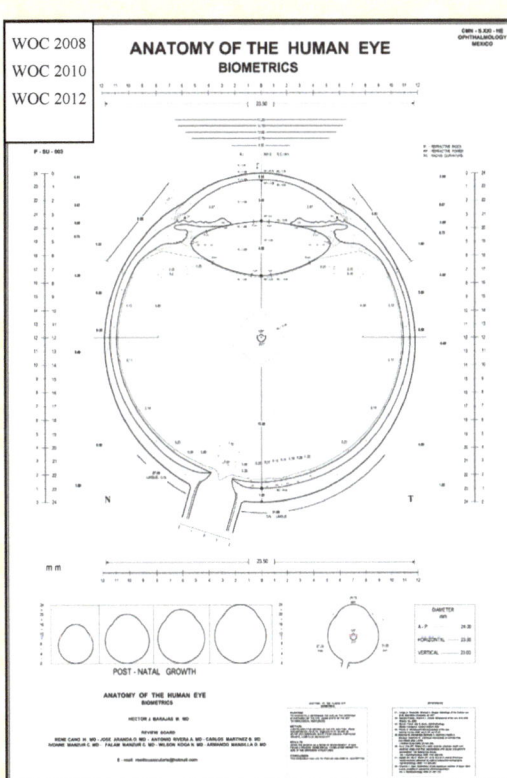

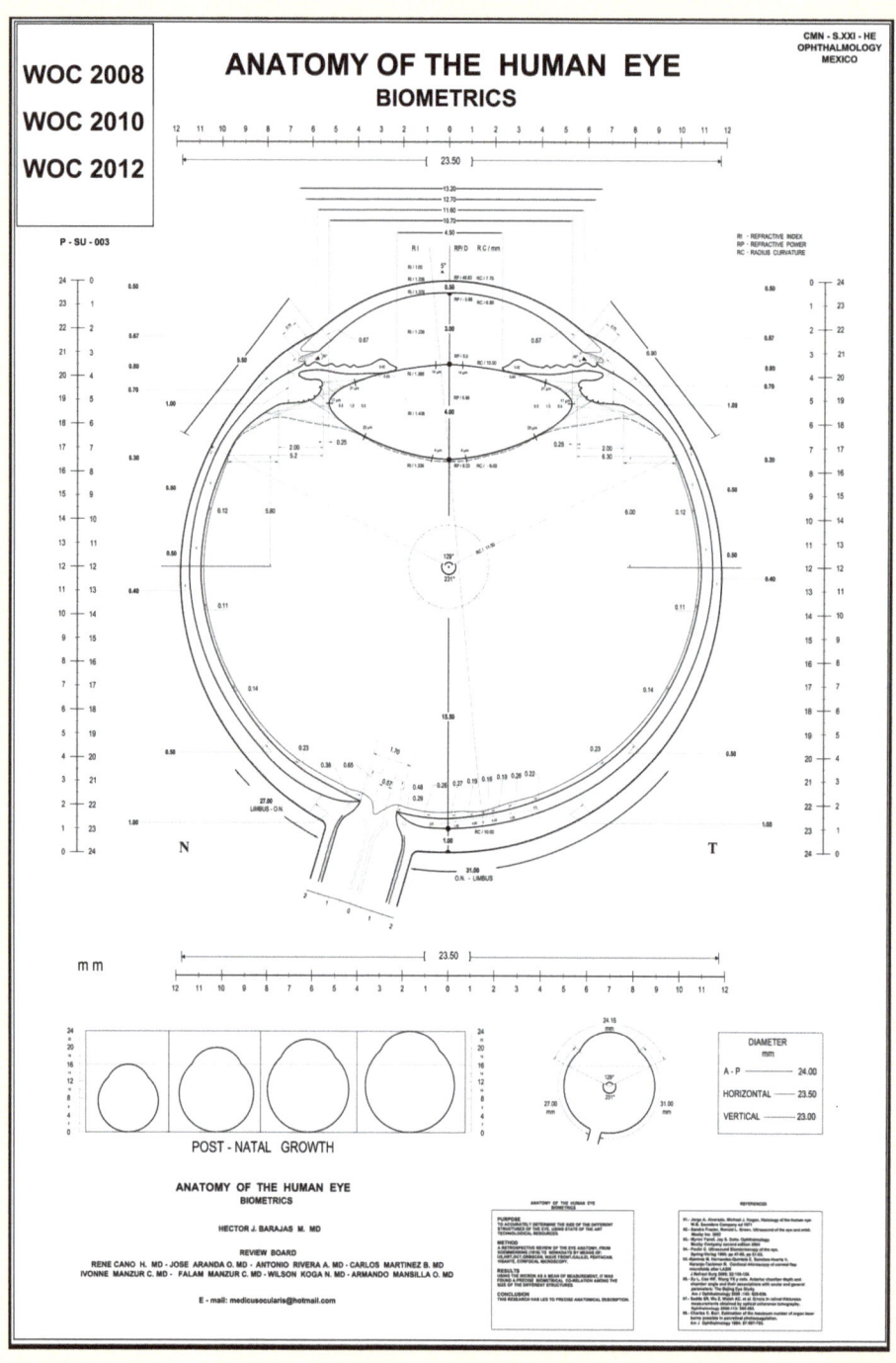

ANATOMY OF THE HUMAN EYE
BIOMETRICS

REFERENCES

01.- Alvarado Jorge A , Michael J. Hogan, Weddell Joan Esperson.

Histology of the human eye. W.B. Saunders Company ed 1971.

02.- Arnaldez, Massignon y Youschkevitch. La science arabe. Paris: PUF 1966.

03.- Barajas H, Aranda J, Rivera A, Martinez C. Manzur I, Manzur F, Koga W,Mansilla A.

The human eye anatomy.   Clinical Experimental Ophthalmology 2008 ; 36 suppl. 305.

04.- Bartish,G. Augendienst 1583, Benevenutus Grassus of Jerusalem . De oculus

Ferrara 1474, Walter Bayley . A brief treatise touching of preservation of the eie sight London :1586 (facsimil).

05.- Binkhorst R. The accuracy of ultrasonic measurement of the axial length of the eye.

Ophthalmic Surg 1981; 12:363-365.

06.-Bruno Halioua,Bernard Ziskind. Medicine in the days of the pharaohs.

The Belknap Press of Harvard University Press   2005.

07.- Buehl W, Danijela S. Comparison of three methods of measuring   corneal thickness and anterior chamber depth. Am J Ophthalmol 2006; 141:7-12.

08.- Charles C. Barr. Estimation of the maximum number of argon laser burns possible in panretinal photocoagulation. American Journal of Ophthalmology 1984; 97:697-703.

09.- Cid Felipe. Historia de la ciencia. Barcelona, España. Ed.Planeta 1977

10.- Claton, M. Leonardo da Vinci. The Anatomy of Man .Boston: Little Brown 1992.

11.- Dada T, Sihota R. Comparison of anterior segment optical coherence tomography and ultrasoundbiomicroscopy for assessment of the anterior segment. J Cataract Refract Surg 2007; 33:837-840.

12.- Dada T, Gadia Ritu, et. al. Anterior segment, imaging in ophthalmology. New Delhi, India: Jaypee brothers, first edition 2008

13.- Enciclopedia Italiana di Scienze. Lettere, de Arti. Roma Istituto della Enciclopedia Italiana,1980.

14.- Frazier Sandra , Green Ronald L. Ultrasound of the eye and orbit. Mosby Inc. 2002.

15.- Gil del Rio E. Ôptica fisiològica clìnica. Barcelona :Ed. Toray, S.A 1980.

16.- Gorin George. History of ophthalmology. Wilmington, Delaware: Publish or Perish, inc.1982.

17.- Grom Eduard. Ensayos sobre historia arte y oftalmologia . Caracas . Boletin I.N.D.I.O. 1988.

18.- Hill W, Angeles R, Otani T. *Evaluation of a new IOL Master algorithm to measure axial length. J. Cataract Refract Surg* 2008; 34(6):920-924.

19.- Hirschberg Julius. *The history of ophthalmology. Bonn. Verlag J.P. Wayenborgh* 1982

20.- Hill W, Angeles R, Otani T. *Evaluation of a new IOL Master algorithm to measure axial length. J. Cataract Refract Surg* 2008; 34(6):920-924.

21.- Kalev-Landoy M, Day AC, Cordeiro MF y cols. *Optical coherence tomography in anterior segment imaging Acta ophthalmol Scand* 2007; 85 (4) 427- 430 .

22.- Konstantopoulos A, Hossain P. *Recent advances in ophthalmic anterior segment imaging: a new era for ophthalmic diagnosis?. Br J Ophthalmol* 2007; 91:551-557.

23.-Ovio Giuseppe . *Storia dell'Oculistica. Italia: Ghibaudo-Cuneo* , 1950.

24.- Pansier P. *A brief conspectus on arab ophthalmology. Barcelona :Laboratorios del norte de España Masnou* 1993.

25.- Pavlin C. *Ultrasound Biomicroscopy of the eye . New York, NY: Springer Verlag* 1995.

26 .- Pazzini, A. *Girolamo Fabrizi d'Acquapendente, his Workand his Teaching. Scienza Medica Italica,* 1960.

27.- Piñero DP, Plaza AB, Alió JL. *Anterior segment biometry with 2 imaging technologies:*
Very-high-frequency ultrasound scanning versus optical coherence tomography.
J Cataract Refract Surg 2008; 34:95-102.

28.- Porter, R. *Dizionario Biografico della Storia della Medicina e delle Scienze Naturali. Milano: FMR.* 1989.

29.- Ramirez M, Hernandez-Quintela E, Sanchez-Huerta V, Naranjo-Tackman R.
Confocal microscopy of corneal flap microfolds after LASIK. J Refract Surg 2006; 22:155-8.

30.- Ramirez M, Hernandez-Quintela E, Sanchez-Huerta V, Naranjo-Tackman R.
Confocal microscopy of corneal flap microfolds after LASIK.J Refract Surg 2006; 22:155-158.

31.- Ramirez M, Hernandez-Quintela E, Naranjo-Tackman R. *A comparative confocal microscopy analysis after LASIK with the Intra Lase femtosecond laser vs Hansatome microkeratome. J Refract Surg* 2007; 23:305-307.

32.- Sakata LM y cols. *Assessment of the scleral spur in anterior segment optical coherence tomography images. Arch ophthalmology 2008; 126 (2) :181-185 .*

33.- Sanchez Huerta V, De Wit Carter G. Hernández-Quintela E, Naranjo-Tackman R. Occupational corneal argyrosis in art silver solderers. Cornea 2003 ; 22:7 604-611.

34.- Santodomingo-Rubido J, Mallen E, Gilmartin B, Wolffsohn J. A new non-contact optical device for ocular biometry. Brit J Ophthalmol 2002; 86:458-462.

35.-Scarborough, J. Roman Medicine, Ithaca,New York: Cornell University Press,2a ed. 1976.

36.-Sigurd Ry Andersen.The eye and its diseases in antiquity.

Acta ophthalmologica. Supplement 213 vol 72, Scriptor , Denmark 1994.

37.- Stewart Duke-Elder and Kenneth C. Wybar. System of ophthalmology, vol 2.

London: Henry Kimpton, 1961.

38.- Xu L, Cao WF, Wang YX y cols. Anterior chamber depth and chamber angle and their associations with ocular and general parameters: The Bejing Eye Study. Am. J. Ophthalmology 2008 ;145 (5) : 929-936.

39.- Yanoff Myron , Duker S. Jay. Ophthalmology. Mosby Company 3rd edition 2008.

40.- Yun L, Jun-Heon K. Comparison of anterior chamber depth measurement between orbscan II and ultrasound biomicroscopy. J Refrac Surg 2007; (23).